Blood Type A+ Diet and Meal Plan

3-Week Exercise Plans and Mouth Watering Recipes to Lose Weight the Healthy Way for Blood Type A+

Rosalee Casper

Table of Contents

Introduction

Have you ever wondered why certain foods seem to energize you while others leave you feeling sluggish or unwell? The answer may lie in your blood type. Dr. Peter D'Adamo's groundbreaking research suggests that our blood type not only determines our susceptibility to certain illnesses but also influences how our bodies respond to different foods.

In this comprehensive guide, we delve into the science behind the Blood Type Diet, exploring how the unique characteristics of Blood Type A+ individuals shape their nutritional needs and dietary preferences. Whether you're new to the concept of blood type diets or seeking to optimize your health through personalized nutrition, this book provides the knowledge and tools you need to thrive.

Throughout the pages that follow, we'll uncover the principles of the Blood Type A+ Diet, identifying beneficial foods that support your well-being and those to avoid that may hinder your health goals. From vibrant fruits and vegetables to nourishing grains and lean proteins, you'll discover a wealth of delicious options tailored to your blood type.

But this book is more than just a collection of dietary guidelines. We'll also delve into the practical aspects of meal planning, offering customizable meal plans, cooking tips, and strategies for incorporating exercise and stress management into your lifestyle. Whether you're a seasoned chef or a novice in the kitchen, you'll find inspiration and guidance to create flavorful, nutritious meals that align with your blood type.

As you embark on this journey, remember that the Blood Type A+ Diet is not a one-size-fits-all approach. It's about honoring your body's unique needs and finding the balance that works best for you. With dedication, patience, and a willingness to explore new flavors and habits, you'll embark on a path toward improved health and vitality.

So, whether you're seeking to shed a few pounds, boost your energy levels, or simply embrace a healthier way of eating, join us as we uncover the secrets of the Blood Type A+ Diet and embark on a transformative journey toward optimal health and wellness.

Let's begin!

Understanding Blood Type A+

What is Blood Type A+?

The ABO blood typing system, discovered by Austrian scientist Karl Landsteiner in the early 20th century, categorizes blood into four main groups: A, B, AB, and O. These groups are determined by the presence or absence of specific antigens – A and B antigens – on the surface of red blood cells. Blood type A individuals have A antigens, blood type B individuals have B antigens, blood type AB individuals have both A and B antigens, and blood type O individuals have neither A nor B antigens.

In addition to the ABO blood group system, blood is also classified based on the presence or absence of the Rh antigen, also known as the Rh factor. The Rh factor is either present (+) or absent (-), resulting in positive or negative blood types. Blood type A+ individuals have both A antigens and the Rh antigen on their red blood cells.

Individuals with blood type A+ share certain characteristics and traits that distinguish them from other blood types. While blood type does not solely determine personality or behavior, some studies suggest that certain traits may be more common among individuals with specific blood types.

Blood type A+ individuals are often described as compassionate, analytical, and detail-oriented. They may thrive in environments that require organization and structure, and they tend to be conscientious and reliable individuals.

Blood type is inherited from our parents through a combination of genetic factors. The ABO blood group system is determined by the presence of specific alleles – variations of a gene – inherited from both parents. For example, a person with blood type A+ may have inherited one A allele from one parent and one O allele from the other parent. The Rh factor, on the other hand, is determined by a separate gene known as the RHD gene. A person with blood type A+ has inherited both the A allele and the Rh-positive allele.

Blood type A+ is one of the most common blood types worldwide, with a prevalence that varies among different populations. In the United States, approximately 34% of the population has blood type A+, making it the second most common blood type after O+. However, the distribution of blood types may differ in other regions and ethnic groups.

Characteristics of Blood Type A+ Individuals

Blood type A+ individuals possess unique characteristics that set them apart from other blood types. While individual traits can vary widely among people, there are some common tendencies associated with this blood type that have been observed through research and anecdotal evidence.

Compassionate and Empathetic

Blood type A+ individuals are often described as compassionate and empathetic. They have a strong sense of empathy and are deeply attuned to the emotions and needs of others. This empathy extends to both humans and animals, as they are often drawn to causes that promote kindness and social justice. Their compassionate nature makes them natural caretakers and advocates for those in need.

Analytical and Detail-Oriented

Individuals with blood type A+ tend to have a meticulous and analytical approach to life. They thrive in environments that require attention to detail and careful planning. Whether it's organizing their workspace or tackling complex problems, they excel at breaking tasks down into manageable steps and analyzing each component thoroughly. This analytical mindset serves them well in professions that demand precision and accuracy, such as accounting, research, or engineering.

Conscientious and Responsible

Blood type A+ individuals are known for their conscientiousness and reliability. They take their commitments seriously and strive to fulfill their obligations to the best of their abilities. Whether it's meeting deadlines at work or supporting loved ones in times of need, they can be counted on to follow through with their promises. Their sense of responsibility extends to their own well-being, as they prioritize self-care and strive to maintain a healthy lifestyle.

Creative and Artistic

Despite their analytical nature, blood type A+ individuals also possess a creative and artistic side. They often have a keen appreciation for beauty and aesthetics, whether it's expressed through visual arts, music, or literature. Many blood type A+ individuals find solace and inspiration in creative pursuits, using them as a means of self-expression and personal growth. Their creativity adds depth and richness to their lives, allowing them to explore new ideas and perspectives.

Sensitivity to Stress

One challenge that blood type A+ individuals may face is a heightened sensitivity to stress. Due to their empathetic nature and tendency towards perfectionism, they may be more susceptible to feelings of anxiety and overwhelm. It's important for blood type A+ individuals to practice self-care and stress management techniques to maintain their emotional well-being. This may include activities such as meditation, yoga, or spending time in nature to recharge and rejuvenate.

Relationship between Blood Type and Diet

The relationship between blood type and diet can be traced back to our evolutionary origins. As humans migrated and adapted to different environments, their diets diversified based on the availability of local resources. This led to the emergence of distinct dietary patterns among different populations, shaped by factors such as climate, geography, and cultural practices.

Genetic Factors

Our blood type is determined by our genetic makeup, specifically the presence or absence of certain antigens on the surface of red blood cells. These genetic factors not only influence our blood type but also play a role in determining how our bodies metabolize and utilize nutrients from food. For example, individuals with blood type A may have inherited genetic traits that favor a plant-based diet, while those with blood type O may have genetic adaptations suited to a more protein-rich diet.

Impact on Digestion and Health

The relationship between blood type and diet extends beyond genetics to encompass how our bodies digest and metabolize different foods. According to the Blood Type Diet theory, certain foods contain lectins – proteins found in foods – that may react differently with the antigens present in our blood, leading to varying degrees of inflammation, digestive discomfort, and other health issues. By aligning our diet with our blood type, proponents of the Blood Type Diet believe we can optimize digestion, enhance nutrient absorption, and reduce the risk of chronic diseases.

Personalized Nutrition

One of the key principles of the Blood Type Diet is personalized nutrition, which emphasizes tailoring dietary choices to individual blood types. By identifying which foods are beneficial, neutral, or detrimental based on their blood type, individuals can optimize their health and well-being. For example, individuals with blood type A may thrive on a predominantly plant-based diet rich in fruits, vegetables, and whole grains, while those with blood type O may benefit from a diet higher in lean protein and limited in grains and dairy.

Chapter 1. How Blood Type A+ Influences Diet

Genetic Factors and Blood Type

Genetic factors play a fundamental role in determining an individual's blood type, which is inherited from their parents according to specific inheritance patterns. The ABO blood group system is governed by multiple alleles – variations of a gene – that determine the presence or absence of A and B antigens on the surface of red blood cells. For example, individuals with blood type A inherit one A allele from one parent and either another A allele or an O allele from the other parent.

Role of Antigens

Antigens are molecules present on the surface of red blood cells that determine blood type. The A and B antigens are glycoproteins that are synthesized by specific enzymes encoded by the ABO gene. The presence or absence of these antigens, along with the presence or absence of the Rh antigen, determines an individual's blood type.

Genetic Variants and Blood Type

Genetic variations in the ABO gene can result in different blood types among individuals. For example, individuals with blood type A have the A antigen on their red blood cells due to the presence of the A allele, while individuals with blood type B have the B antigen due to the presence of the B allele. Similarly, individuals with blood type O lack both A and B antigens due to the presence of two O alleles.

Rh Factor

In addition to the ABO blood group system, blood type is also influenced by the presence or absence of the Rh antigen, also known as the Rh factor. The Rh factor is determined by a separate gene known as the RHD gene. Individuals who inherit the Rh antigen from one or both parents are classified as Rh-positive (e.g., A+, B+), while those who do not inherit the Rh antigen are classified as Rh-negative (e.g., A-, B-).

Implications for Nutrition and Health

Genetic factors associated with blood type can influence various aspects of nutrition and health. For example, individuals with blood type A may have genetic predispositions that favor a plant-based diet rich in fruits, vegetables, and whole grains, while individuals with blood type O may have genetic adaptations suited to a more protein-rich diet. By understanding how genetic factors intersect with blood type, it is possible to tailor dietary recommendations to better meet individual nutritional needs and promote optimal health.

Role of Lectins in Food Compatibility

Lectins are carbohydrate-binding proteins found in a wide range of plant foods, including grains, legumes, fruits, and vegetables. They serve various functions in plants, such as seed germination, defense against pests, and modulation of microbial populations in the soil. While lectins are abundant in many foods, their levels and effects can vary depending on factors such as food processing, cooking methods, and individual tolerance.

Interaction with Blood Type Antigens

One of the key concepts of the Blood Type Diet is that lectins can interact with specific blood type antigens present on the surface of red blood cells, potentially influencing metabolic responses and immune reactions. For example, individuals with blood type A may be more sensitive to lectins found in certain grains and legumes, while individuals with blood type O may be better able to tolerate these foods.

Beneficial and Detrimental Lectins

Not all lectins are created equal when it comes to their effects on health. While some lectins may have beneficial effects, such as promoting gut health and modulating immune function, others may be detrimental, contributing to inflammation and digestive issues. The Blood Type Diet aims to identify and prioritize foods that contain beneficial lectins for each blood type while minimizing exposure to potentially harmful lectins.

Food Compatibility Based on Blood Type

By considering the interactions between lectins and blood type antigens, the Blood Type Diet offers personalized recommendations for food compatibility tailored to each blood type. For example, individuals with blood type A may be advised to prioritize plant-based foods such as fruits, vegetables, and whole grains, which contain lectins that are more compatible with their blood type. Conversely, individuals with blood type O may be encouraged to focus on protein-rich foods such as lean meats and seafood, which are less likely to contain lectins that are incompatible with their blood type.

Impact on Digestion and Health

One of the central tenets of the Blood Type Diet is that certain foods may be more or less compatible with an individual's blood type, influencing digestion and nutrient absorption. For example, individuals with blood type A may be advised to prioritize plant-based foods, which are believed to be more easily digested and metabolized, while individuals with blood type O may benefit from a higher protein intake, which may support optimal digestion and energy levels.

Inflammatory Responses

The Blood Type Diet suggests that dietary choices based on blood type can help reduce inflammation and promote overall health. Certain foods, particularly those containing lectins that are incompatible with an individual's blood type, may trigger inflammatory responses and contribute to symptoms such as bloating, gas, and discomfort. By avoiding or minimizing exposure to these inflammatory foods, individuals may experience improvements in digestive health and overall well-being.

Nutrient Absorption

Optimal digestion is essential for efficient nutrient absorption, which plays a critical role in supporting overall health and vitality. The Blood Type Diet proposes that aligning dietary choices with an individual's blood type can enhance nutrient absorption and utilization, leading to improvements in energy levels, immune function, and metabolic processes. For example, individuals with blood type A may benefit from a diet rich in plant-based foods, which provide essential vitamins, minerals, and antioxidants necessary for optimal health.

Gut Microbiota

The gut microbiota, comprised of trillions of microorganisms that inhabit the digestive tract, plays a crucial role in digestion, immune function, and overall health. The Blood Type Diet suggests that dietary choices based on blood type may influence the composition and diversity of the gut microbiota, leading to improvements in digestive health and immune function. By consuming foods that are compatible with their blood type, individuals may support a healthy balance of gut bacteria and reduce the risk of gastrointestinal issues.

Weight Management

The Blood Type Diet proposes that personalized dietary recommendations based on blood type can support weight management and body composition goals. By aligning dietary choices with an individual's genetic predispositions and metabolic processes, the diet aims to optimize energy balance and promote sustainable weight loss or maintenance. For example, individuals with blood type O may be encouraged to focus on lean protein sources and limit refined carbohydrates to support healthy weight management and metabolic function.

Overall Well-being

Ultimately, the goal of the Blood Type Diet is to promote overall well-being by optimizing digestion, supporting nutrient absorption, reducing inflammation, and maintaining a healthy weight. By tailoring dietary choices to an individual's blood type, the diet aims to address underlying genetic factors that may influence digestive health and overall health outcomes. While further research is needed to fully elucidate the mechanisms underlying the diet's effects on digestion and health, many individuals report improvements in digestive symptoms, energy levels, and overall quality of life when following the principles of the Blood Type Diet.

Chapter 2. Key Food Groups for Blood Type A+

Fruits and Vegetables

Fruits and vegetables are nutrient-dense foods that provide a wide array of essential vitamins, minerals, and phytonutrients necessary for optimal health. They are rich sources of vitamin C, vitamin A, potassium, folate, and dietary fiber, among other nutrients, which support immune function, heart health, digestion, and overall well-being. By incorporating a variety of colorful fruits and vegetables into their diets, individuals can ensure they receive a diverse range of nutrients necessary for optimal health.

Antioxidant Content

Many fruits and vegetables are rich in antioxidants, which help protect cells from damage caused by oxidative stress and free radicals. Antioxidants such as vitamin C, vitamin E, beta-carotene, and flavonoids have been shown to reduce inflammation, support cardiovascular health, and reduce the risk of chronic diseases such as cancer and Alzheimer's disease. By consuming antioxidant-rich fruits and vegetables, individuals can support their body's natural defense mechanisms and promote long-term health and vitality.

Fiber Content

Fruits and vegetables are excellent sources of dietary fiber, which is essential for promoting digestive health, regulating blood sugar levels, and supporting weight management. Fiber helps to bulk up stool, promote regular bowel movements, and nourish beneficial gut bacteria, which contribute to improved digestion and reduced risk of gastrointestinal issues such as constipation, diverticulosis, and irritable bowel syndrome (IBS). By including fiber-rich fruits and vegetables in their diets, individuals can support optimal digestive function and overall well-being.

Healing Properties

Certain fruits and vegetables recommended for specific blood types are believed to possess unique healing properties that can promote health and well-being. For example, individuals with blood type A+ may benefit from consuming alkaline-forming fruits and vegetables such as berries, apples, broccoli, and spinach, which help balance acidity levels in the body and support immune function. By selecting fruits and vegetables tailored to their blood type, individuals can optimize their nutrient intake and support their body's natural healing processes.

Variety and Seasonality

Incorporating a variety of fruits and vegetables into the diet ensures individuals receive a diverse range of nutrients and phytonutrients necessary for optimal health. It is important to include a rainbow of colors, textures, and flavors in meals and snacks to maximize nutrient intake and promote overall well-being. Additionally, choosing fruits and vegetables that are in season and locally grown can enhance flavor, freshness, and nutritional value, while also supporting environmental sustainability.

Whole Grains and Legumes

Whole grains and legumes are rich sources of complex carbohydrates, which provide sustained energy and support stable blood sugar levels. Unlike refined grains, which are stripped of their bran and germ during processing, whole grains retain their fiber-rich outer layer, providing a slow and steady release of energy. Complex carbohydrates help to fuel physical activity, support cognitive function, and prevent energy crashes and sugar cravings.

Dietary Fiber

Whole grains and legumes are excellent sources of dietary fiber, which is essential for promoting digestive health, regulating bowel movements, and supporting weight management. Fiber helps to bulk up stool, promote feelings of fullness and satiety, and nourish beneficial gut bacteria, which contribute to improved digestion and reduced risk of gastrointestinal issues such as constipation, diverticulosis, and hemorrhoids.

Protein Content

Legumes are rich sources of plant-based protein, which is essential for supporting muscle growth and repair, immune function, hormone production, and satiety. Whole grains also contain some protein, although in smaller quantities compared to legumes. By incorporating a variety of whole grains and legumes into their diets, individuals can meet their daily protein needs and support overall health and well-being.

Vitamins and Minerals

Whole grains and legumes are rich sources of vitamins and minerals, including B vitamins, iron, magnesium, zinc, and phosphorus, which are essential for supporting various physiological functions in the body. B vitamins play critical roles in energy metabolism, nerve function, and red blood cell production, while minerals such as iron and magnesium are involved in oxygen transport, muscle function, and bone health.

Antioxidant and Anti-inflammatory Properties

Certain whole grains and legumes contain antioxidants and anti-inflammatory compounds that help protect cells from damage caused by oxidative stress and reduce inflammation in the body. For example, whole grains such as oats, quinoa, and brown rice contain antioxidants such as tocopherols, polyphenols, and lignans, which have been shown to reduce inflammation, lower cholesterol levels, and support heart health.

Gluten-Free Options

For individuals with gluten sensitivity or celiac disease, gluten-containing grains such as wheat, barley, and rye should be avoided or minimized. Fortunately, there are many gluten-free whole grains and legumes available that can provide similar nutritional benefits without triggering adverse reactions. Gluten-free options include quinoa, brown rice, buckwheat, millet, amaranth, chickpeas, lentils, and black beans, which can be incorporated into meals and snacks to support a gluten-free lifestyle.

Lean Proteins and Dairy Alternatives

Lean proteins are rich sources of high-quality protein, which is essential for supporting muscle growth and repair, immune function, hormone production, and satiety. Lean protein sources include poultry, fish, seafood, tofu, tempeh, seitan, and legumes, which provide essential amino acids necessary for optimal health. By incorporating lean proteins into their diets, individuals can meet their daily protein needs and support overall health and well-being.

Omega-3 Fatty Acids

Certain lean protein sources, such as fatty fish like salmon, trout, and sardines, are rich in omega-3 fatty acids, which have been shown to support heart health, brain function, and inflammation regulation. Omega-3 fatty acids are essential fats that must be obtained through diet, as the body cannot produce them on its own. By including omega-3-rich lean proteins in their diets, individuals can support cardiovascular health, cognitive function, and overall well-being.

Plant-Based Protein Alternatives

For individuals following plant-based or vegetarian diets, plant-based protein alternatives such as tofu, tempeh, seitan, legumes, and soy products can provide excellent sources of protein and essential nutrients. These plant-based protein sources are rich in fiber, vitamins, minerals, and phytonutrients, which support digestive health, immune function, and overall well-being. By incorporating a variety of plant-based protein alternatives into their diets, individuals can meet their nutritional needs and support their dietary preferences.

Dairy Alternatives

For individuals with lactose intolerance, dairy allergies, or those following vegan diets, dairy alternatives such as almond milk, soy milk, coconut milk, oat milk, and rice milk can provide nutritious alternatives to traditional dairy products. These dairy alternatives are often fortified with vitamins and minerals such as calcium, vitamin D, and vitamin B12 to provide similar nutritional benefits to dairy milk. By choosing dairy alternatives that are compatible with their blood type, individuals can enjoy the taste and versatility of dairy products without experiencing adverse reactions.

Calcium and Vitamin D

Dairy products and dairy alternatives are important sources of calcium and vitamin D, which are essential for supporting bone health, muscle function, and overall well-being. Calcium is necessary for building and maintaining strong bones and teeth, while vitamin D helps regulate calcium absorption and utilization in the body. By incorporating calcium-rich dairy products or dairy alternatives into their diets, individuals can support their bone health and reduce the risk of osteoporosis and fractures.

Moderation and Balance

While lean proteins and dairy alternatives can provide valuable nutrients and health benefits, it is important to consume them in moderation and balance within the context of a varied and balanced diet. Too much protein, especially from animal sources, can strain the kidneys and contribute to increased risk of chronic diseases such as heart disease and kidney disease. Similarly, consuming excessive amounts of dairy or dairy alternatives may contribute to excess calorie intake and potential nutrient imbalances. By practicing moderation and balance, individuals can enjoy the benefits of lean proteins and dairy alternatives while supporting overall health and well-being.

Chapter 3. Common Foods to Eliminate

Processed Meats and Sugary Snacks

Processed meats are meats that have been preserved by curing, smoking, salting, or adding preservatives. These meats often contain high levels of unhealthy fats, sodium, nitrates, and other additives, which can contribute to inflammation, heart disease, and other health issues. Common processed meats include bacon, sausage, hot dogs, deli meats, and canned meats.

Sugary Snacks

Sugary snacks are foods that contain high levels of added sugars, such as candy, cookies, cakes, pastries, soda, and sweetened beverages. These foods are often high in calories, low in nutrients, and lacking in fiber, protein, and healthy fats, leading to rapid spikes and crashes in blood sugar levels. Consuming sugary snacks regularly can contribute to weight gain, insulin resistance, type 2 diabetes, and other metabolic disorders.

Moderation and Balance

While processed meats and sugary snacks are generally discouraged in the Blood Type Diet, occasional indulgences can be enjoyed in moderation as part of a balanced diet. By prioritizing whole, nutrient-dense foods and limiting processed meats and sugary snacks, individuals can support their health and well-being and reduce the risk of adverse health effects associated with these foods.

Dairy Products and Fatty Foods

Dairy products include milk, cheese, yogurt, butter, and cream, among others. While dairy products are excellent sources of calcium, protein, and other essential nutrients, they may also pose challenges for some individuals due to lactose intolerance, allergies, or sensitivities. Additionally, dairy products can be high in saturated fat, which has been linked to increased cholesterol levels and heart disease risk.

Potential Issues

For individuals with lactose intolerance or dairy allergies, consuming dairy products can lead to digestive discomfort, bloating, gas, diarrhea, and other gastrointestinal symptoms. Additionally, some individuals may be sensitive to the proteins found in dairy, such as casein and whey, which can trigger inflammatory responses and immune reactions. Even for individuals without lactose intolerance or allergies, consuming high amounts of dairy products may contribute to excess calorie intake and weight gain due to their high fat and calorie content.

Fatty Foods

Fatty foods include foods that are high in unhealthy fats, such as saturated fats and trans fats. These fats are commonly found in fried foods, processed foods, fatty meats, full-fat dairy products, and certain oils (such as palm oil and coconut oil). Consuming high amounts of fatty foods can contribute to weight gain, elevated cholesterol levels, heart disease, and other health issues.

Health Risks

Eating too many fatty foods, particularly those high in saturated and trans fats, can increase levels of LDL cholesterol (often referred to as "bad" cholesterol) in the blood, which can contribute to atherosclerosis (hardening of the arteries) and increase the risk of heart disease and stroke. Additionally, fatty foods are often high in calories and low in essential nutrients, leading to excess calorie intake, weight gain, and nutrient deficiencies.

High-Glycemic Index Carbohydrates

The glycemic index (GI) is a measure of how quickly carbohydrates in foods raise blood sugar levels after consumption. Foods with a high GI are rapidly digested and absorbed, causing a rapid spike in blood sugar levels, followed by a subsequent crash. High-glycemic index carbohydrates are often refined carbohydrates that have been processed and stripped of their natural fiber and nutrients, such as white bread, white rice, sugary cereals, and baked goods made with white flour.

Effects on Blood Sugar Levels

Consuming high-glycemic index carbohydrates can lead to rapid fluctuations in blood sugar levels, which can negatively impact energy levels, mood, and cognitive function. The rapid rise in blood sugar levels triggers the release of insulin, a hormone that helps cells absorb glucose from the bloodstream. However, excessive insulin release can lead to a rapid drop in blood sugar levels, causing feelings of fatigue, irritability, and cravings for more sugary foods.

Health Risks

Repeated spikes and crashes in blood sugar levels can contribute to insulin resistance, a condition in which cells become less responsive to insulin, leading to elevated blood sugar levels and an increased risk of type 2 diabetes. Additionally, high-glycemic index carbohydrates have been associated with weight gain, obesity, heart disease, and other metabolic disorders. Consuming high amounts of refined carbohydrates can also lead to inflammation, oxidative stress, and other adverse health effects.

Blood Type Considerations

In the Blood Type Diet, individuals with specific blood types may be more sensitive to high-glycemic index carbohydrates, leading to adverse reactions such as weight gain, fatigue, and digestive discomfort. For example, individuals with blood type A may be advised to limit consumption of high-glycemic index carbohydrates such as white bread, white rice, and sugary snacks, which can contribute to blood sugar imbalances and other health issues.

Moderation and Balance

While high-glycemic index carbohydrates should be limited in the diet, they can still be enjoyed occasionally as part of a balanced meal or snack. By pairing high-glycemic index carbohydrates with protein, fiber, and healthy fats, individuals can help slow down the absorption of glucose into the bloodstream and minimize the impact on blood sugar levels. Additionally, portion control and mindful eating practices can help prevent overconsumption of high-glycemic index carbohydrates and promote overall health and well-being.

Chapter 4. Building Blocks of a Balanced Diet

Macronutrient Ratios

Protein

Protein is an essential macronutrient that plays a vital role in building and repairing tissues, supporting immune function, and providing energy. The ideal protein intake may vary depending on factors such as age, gender, activity level, and health status. In the Blood Type Diet, individuals are advised to consume high-quality sources of protein tailored to their blood type. For example, individuals with blood type O may benefit from a higher intake of animal-based proteins such as lean meats, poultry, and fish, while individuals with blood type A may thrive on plant-based protein sources such as legumes, tofu, and tempeh.

Carbohydrates

Carbohydrates are the body's primary source of energy and play a crucial role in fueling metabolic processes, supporting brain function, and maintaining blood sugar levels. The ideal carbohydrate intake may vary depending on factors such as activity level, metabolic rate, and blood sugar regulation. In the Blood Type Diet, individuals are encouraged to focus on complex carbohydrates that provide sustained energy and promote stable blood sugar levels. For example, individuals with blood type A may benefit from a higher intake of whole grains, fruits, and vegetables, while individuals with blood type O may thrive on a lower-carbohydrate, higher-protein diet.

Fat

Fat is an essential macronutrient that plays a crucial role in hormone production, cell membrane integrity, and nutrient absorption. The ideal fat intake may vary depending on factors such as metabolic rate, hormone balance, and cardiovascular health. In the Blood Type Diet, individuals are advised to focus on healthy fats that provide essential fatty acids and support overall health and well-being. For example, individuals with blood type A may benefit from a higher intake of plant-based fats such as avocados, nuts, and seeds, while individuals with blood type O may thrive on a diet rich in omega-3 fatty acids found in fatty fish, flaxseeds, and walnuts.

Portion Control Guidelines

Portion control plays a crucial role in maintaining a healthy weight, managing blood sugar levels, and supporting overall health. Consuming appropriate portion sizes helps prevent overeating, regulates calorie intake, and promotes a balanced distribution of macronutrients. By practicing portion control, individuals can avoid excessive calorie consumption, reduce the risk of weight gain and obesity-related health issues, and support their long-term health goals.

Tailoring Portions to Blood Type

In the Blood Type Diet, portion control guidelines are tailored to individual blood types, taking into account factors such as metabolic rate, energy needs, and nutrient requirements. For example, individuals with blood type O, who are often advised to follow a higher-protein, lower-carbohydrate diet, may benefit from larger portions of lean proteins such as poultry, fish, and lean cuts of meat, while individuals with blood type A, who are encouraged to focus on plant-based foods, may benefit from larger portions of fruits, vegetables, and whole grains.

Practical Tips for Portion Control

Practicing portion control doesn't have to be complicated. Simple strategies such as using smaller plates and bowls, measuring serving sizes with kitchen tools or visual cues, and being mindful of hunger and satiety cues can help individuals regulate portion sizes and prevent overeating. Additionally, pre-portioning meals and snacks, avoiding eating straight from packages, and focusing on nutrient-dense foods can support portion control and promote healthier eating habits.

Monitoring and Adjusting

Monitoring portion sizes and adjusting as needed based on individual needs and goals is essential for long-term success. Regularly assessing portion sizes, energy levels, hunger cues, and weight management can help individuals fine-tune their portion control strategies and achieve optimal results. By staying attuned to their body's needs and making adjustments as necessary, individuals can support their health and well-being and maintain a balanced approach to eating.

Incorporating Mindful Eating

In addition to portion control, practicing mindful eating can further support overall health and well-being. Mindful eating involves paying attention to the sensory experience of eating, including taste, texture, aroma, and satiety cues. By slowing down, savoring each bite, and being present in the moment during meals, individuals can enhance their enjoyment of food, promote digestion, and foster a healthier relationship with food.

Meal Timing and Frequency

Meal timing refers to the schedule of when meals and snacks are consumed throughout the day. Proper meal timing helps regulate hunger and satiety cues, stabilize blood sugar levels, and optimize energy levels. By aligning meal timing with individual circadian rhythms and metabolic needs, individuals can support metabolic efficiency, promote digestion, and enhance overall health and well-being.

Tailoring Meal Timing to Blood Type

In the Blood Type Diet, meal timing recommendations are tailored to individual blood types, taking into account factors such as metabolic rate, energy needs, and nutrient requirements. For example, individuals with blood type O, who are often advised to follow a higher-protein, lower-carbohydrate diet, may benefit from consuming larger meals earlier in the day to support energy levels and promote satiety. Conversely, individuals with blood type A, who are encouraged to focus on plant-based foods, may benefit from smaller, more frequent meals to maintain stable blood sugar levels and prevent energy dips.

Breakfast

Breakfast is often referred to as the most important meal of the day, setting the tone for energy levels, metabolism, and cognitive function. Consuming a balanced breakfast within an hour or two of waking helps kickstart metabolism, stabilize blood sugar levels, and provide essential nutrients to fuel the body and brain. In the Blood Type Diet, breakfast recommendations may vary depending on individual blood types, with emphasis on nutrient-dense foods that support metabolic efficiency and promote overall well-being.

Lunch and Dinner

Lunch and dinner provide opportunities to replenish energy stores, satisfy hunger, and nourish the body with essential nutrients. In the Blood Type Diet, lunch and dinner recommendations may include a balance of lean proteins, complex carbohydrates, and healthy fats tailored to individual blood types. By incorporating a variety of nutrient-dense foods and paying attention to portion sizes, individuals can support optimal energy levels, digestion, and overall health.

Snacks

Snacks can help bridge the gap between meals, regulate hunger and satiety cues, and prevent overeating at mealtime. In the Blood Type Diet, snack recommendations may vary depending on individual blood types and nutritional needs. Healthy snack options may include fruits, vegetables, nuts, seeds, yogurt, and whole-grain crackers, providing a balance of carbohydrates, protein, and fats to support sustained energy and promote satiety.

Chapter 5. Sample Meal Plans

Breakfast, Lunch, Dinner, and Snack Ideas

Breakfast Ideas:

1. Avocado Toast: Top whole-grain toast with mashed avocado, sliced tomatoes, and a sprinkle of sea salt and black pepper.

2. Greek Yogurt Parfait: Layer Greek yogurt with mixed berries, granola, and a drizzle of honey or maple syrup.

3. Veggie Omelette: Whip up an omelette with sautéed vegetables such as spinach, mushrooms, and bell peppers, topped with a sprinkle of cheese.

4. Overnight Oats: Mix rolled oats with almond milk, chia seeds, and a dash of vanilla extract, then refrigerate overnight and top with sliced fruit and nuts in the morning.

5. Smoothie Bowl: Blend frozen banana, spinach, almond milk, and protein powder, then top with sliced fruit, nuts, seeds, and a drizzle of nut butter.

6. Quinoa Breakfast Bowl: Cook quinoa in coconut milk, then top with sliced bananas, toasted coconut flakes, and a dollop of Greek yogurt.

7. Breakfast Burrito: Fill a whole-grain tortilla with scrambled eggs, black beans, salsa, avocado, and a sprinkle of cheese.

8. Peanut Butter Banana Toast: Spread peanut butter on whole-grain toast and top with sliced bananas and a sprinkle of cinnamon.

9. Chia Seed Pudding: Mix chia seeds with almond milk and a touch of honey, then refrigerate until thickened and top with fresh berries.

10. Cottage Cheese and Fruit: Pair cottage cheese with mixed fruit such as pineapple, mango, and kiwi for a refreshing and protein-rich breakfast.

Lunch Ideas:

1. Quinoa Salad: Combine cooked quinoa with chopped cucumbers, tomatoes, avocado, and feta cheese, dressed with lemon vinaigrette.

2. Chickpea Salad Wrap: Fill a whole-grain wrap with chickpea salad, mixed greens, shredded carrots, and hummus.

3. Turkey and Avocado Wrap: Wrap sliced turkey breast, avocado, lettuce, and tomato in a whole-grain tortilla, and drizzle with Greek yogurt dressing.

4. Veggie Stir-Fry: Stir-fry tofu or tempeh with broccoli, bell peppers, snap peas, and carrots in a teriyaki sauce, served over brown rice.

5. Lentil Soup: Simmer lentils with carrots, celery, onions, and tomatoes in vegetable broth, seasoned with cumin, paprika, and coriander.

6. Caprese Salad: Layer sliced tomatoes, fresh mozzarella, and basil leaves on a plate, drizzle with balsamic glaze, and sprinkle with sea salt and black pepper.

7. Grilled Chicken Salad: Grill chicken breast and serve over mixed greens with cherry tomatoes, cucumbers, and sliced almonds, dressed with balsamic vinaigrette.

8. Tuna Salad Lettuce Wraps: Mix canned tuna with Greek yogurt, diced celery, and lemon juice, then scoop onto lettuce leaves and roll up.

9. Quinoa Veggie Bowl: Top cooked quinoa with roasted vegetables, chickpeas, feta cheese, and a squeeze of lemon juice.

10. Turkey and Hummus Sandwich: Spread hummus on whole-grain bread, layer with sliced turkey, cucumber, lettuce, and sprouts.

Dinner Ideas:

1. Baked Salmon with Roasted Vegetables: Season salmon fillets with lemon juice, garlic, and dill, then bake and serve with roasted broccoli, cauliflower, and carrots.

2. Stir-Fried Tofu with Brown Rice: Stir-fry tofu with mixed vegetables in a ginger soy sauce, and serve over cooked brown rice.

3. Spaghetti Squash with Marinara Sauce: Roast spaghetti squash and toss with marinara sauce, sautéed mushrooms, and fresh basil.

4. Grilled Chicken with Quinoa Pilaf: Grill chicken breast and serve with quinoa pilaf cooked with onions, garlic, and mixed vegetables.

5. Veggie Stir-Fry with Noodles: Stir-fry bell peppers, snap peas, carrots, and tofu in a sesame ginger sauce, and toss with cooked soba noodles.

6. Stuffed Bell Peppers: Fill bell peppers with a mixture of cooked ground turkey, quinoa, black beans, corn, and salsa, then bake until tender.

7. Eggplant Parmesan: Bread eggplant slices, bake until crispy, then layer with marinara sauce and mozzarella cheese, and bake until bubbly.

8. Shrimp and Vegetable Skewers: Thread shrimp, cherry tomatoes, bell peppers, and zucchini onto skewers, grill until cooked through, and serve with quinoa.

9. Lentil Curry with Naan Bread: Simmer lentils, tomatoes, onions, and curry spices in coconut milk, and serve with warm naan bread.

10. Baked Chicken with Sweet Potato Mash: Bake chicken thighs with rosemary and lemon, and serve with mashed sweet potatoes seasoned with cinnamon and nutmeg.

Snack Ideas:

1. Apple Slices with Peanut Butter: Dip apple slices in peanut butter for a satisfying and crunchy snack.

2. Greek Yogurt with Granola: Top Greek yogurt with granola and a drizzle of honey or maple syrup for a sweet and protein-rich snack.

3. Hummus and Veggie Sticks: Dip carrot, celery, and cucumber sticks into hummus for a refreshing and nutritious snack.

4. Trail Mix: Mix together nuts, seeds, dried fruit, and dark chocolate chips for a portable and energizing snack.

5. Cottage Cheese with Pineapple: Pair cottage cheese with fresh pineapple chunks for a protein-packed and tropical snack.

6. Rice Cake with Avocado: Spread mashed avocado on a rice cake and top with sliced tomatoes and a sprinkle of sea salt.

7. Hard-Boiled Eggs: Enjoy hard-boiled eggs sprinkled with paprika or black pepper for a quick and protein-rich snack.

8. Almonds and Dried Apricots: Combine almonds and dried apricots for a satisfying and nutrient-dense snack.

9. Greek Yogurt Bark: Spread Greek yogurt onto a baking sheet, top with mixed berries and a drizzle of honey, then freeze and break into pieces for a frozen treat.

10. Edamame: Enjoy steamed edamame pods sprinkled with sea salt for a protein-packed and satisfying snack.

Adjusting for Dietary Preferences and Allergies

Individuals may have dietary preferences based on cultural, ethical, or personal reasons that influence their food choices. These preferences can include vegetarianism, veganism, pescatarianism, or other dietary patterns. When following the Blood Type Diet, it's important to adapt meal plans to align with these preferences while still meeting nutritional needs.

For example, individuals who prefer a plant-based diet can focus on incorporating more legumes, tofu, tempeh, nuts, seeds, and plant-based protein sources into their meals. They can also explore creative ways to incorporate a variety of fruits, vegetables, whole grains, and plant-based fats to ensure a balanced and nutritious diet.

Food Allergies and Intolerances

Food allergies and intolerances require careful consideration when planning meals and selecting ingredients. Common food allergens include peanuts, tree nuts, dairy, eggs, soy, wheat, fish, and shellfish. Individuals with food allergies or intolerances must avoid these allergens to prevent adverse reactions.

When following the Blood Type Diet, individuals with allergies or intolerances can substitute allergenic foods with suitable alternatives. For example, individuals allergic to dairy can choose plant-based milk alternatives such as almond milk, soy milk, or coconut milk. Those allergic to gluten can opt for gluten-free grains such as quinoa, rice, millet, or buckwheat.

Cross-Contamination and Label Reading

To prevent accidental exposure to allergens, individuals must be vigilant about cross-contamination and carefully read food labels. Cross-contamination can occur when allergenic foods come into contact with non-allergenic foods during preparation, cooking, or serving. It's essential to use separate cooking utensils, cutting boards, and kitchen equipment when preparing allergen-free meals.

Reading food labels is also crucial to identify potential allergens in packaged foods. Ingredients lists and allergen statements can provide information about the presence of common allergens in processed foods. Individuals with allergies should familiarize themselves with food label terminology and be diligent about checking labels for allergen warnings.

Customizing Recipes

Adapting recipes to accommodate dietary preferences and allergies requires creativity and flexibility in the kitchen. Substituting ingredients, adjusting cooking methods, and experimenting with new flavors can help individuals create delicious and nutritious meals that align with their dietary needs.

For example, individuals allergic to eggs can use flax or chia seeds mixed with water as a vegan egg substitute in baking recipes. Those avoiding gluten can use alternative flours such as almond flour, coconut flour, or chickpea flour in place of wheat flour. Similarly, individuals following a vegetarian or vegan diet can modify recipes by swapping animal-based ingredients with plant-based alternatives.

Chapter 6. Cooking Techniques for Blood Type A+

Methods to Maximize Nutrient Retention

Cooking methods that involve gentle heat and minimal water exposure are ideal for preserving the nutritional integrity of foods. Techniques such as steaming, sautéing, and stir-frying require shorter cooking times and minimal liquid, helping to retain vitamins, minerals, and phytonutrients.

Steaming

Steaming is a gentle cooking method that involves cooking foods over boiling water. This technique helps to preserve the color, texture, and nutritional content of vegetables, fish, and other delicate foods. Steaming also minimizes nutrient loss compared to boiling or frying, making it an excellent choice for maximizing nutrient retention.

Sautéing and Stir-Frying

Sautéing and stir-frying involve cooking foods quickly over high heat in a small amount of oil or broth. These methods help to preserve the natural flavors and nutrients of ingredients while creating delicious and nutritious meals. By cooking foods briefly and maintaining their texture and color, sautéing and stir-frying can help maximize nutrient retention.

Quick Cooking

Quick cooking methods such as grilling, broiling, and roasting are effective for retaining nutrients in foods while imparting flavor through caramelization and browning. By cooking foods at high temperatures for short periods, quick cooking methods help to lock in moisture and preserve the nutritional value of ingredients.

Minimal Processing

Minimally processed foods retain more nutrients than heavily processed counterparts. Choosing whole, unprocessed foods whenever possible ensures maximum nutrient retention and promotes optimal health. Foods such as fruits, vegetables, whole grains, lean proteins, and healthy fats provide essential nutrients in their natural forms, supporting overall well-being.

Proper Storage

Proper storage techniques help to maintain the freshness and nutritional quality of foods over time. Storing fruits and vegetables in the refrigerator, in airtight containers, or in the crisper drawer helps to slow down spoilage and preserve their vitamins and minerals. Likewise, storing grains, legumes, nuts, and seeds in a cool, dry place can extend their shelf life and prevent nutrient degradation.

Eating Fresh and Seasonal Foods

Choosing fresh, seasonal produce ensures maximum flavor and nutritional value. Seasonal fruits and vegetables are often harvested at peak ripeness, meaning they contain higher levels of vitamins, minerals, and antioxidants. Incorporating a variety of fresh, seasonal foods into meals supports overall health and provides a diverse array of nutrients.

Flavorful Seasoning Alternatives

Herbs and Spices

Herbs and spices are versatile flavor enhancers that add depth and complexity to dishes without the need for excessive salt or sugar. Experimenting with a variety of herbs and spices allows individuals to create unique flavor profiles tailored to their preferences. Common herbs and spices include:

- Basil
- Cilantro
- Parsley
- Thyme
- Rosemary
- Oregano
- Sage
- Mint
- Paprika
- Cumin
- Turmeric
- Ginger
- Garlic
- Onion powder
- Chili powder

Citrus Zest and Juice

Citrus zest and juice add brightness and acidity to dishes, enhancing flavor and balance. Zesting citrus fruits such as lemons, limes, and oranges adds aromatic oils and intense flavor to sauces, dressings, marinades, and desserts.

Likewise, squeezing fresh citrus juice over grilled meats, roasted vegetables, or salads imparts a refreshing tanginess and elevates the overall taste.

Vinegars

Vinegars are acidic condiments that provide depth and complexity to dishes. Balsamic vinegar, apple cider vinegar, red wine vinegar, and rice vinegar are commonly used in cooking and salad dressings to add acidity and balance. Experimenting with different types of vinegars allows individuals to customize flavors and enhance the taste of their meals.

Aromatics

Aromatics such as onions, garlic, shallots, and scallions provide a strong flavor base for savory dishes. Sautéing aromatics in olive oil or broth releases their natural oils and enhances their sweetness and depth of flavor. Incorporating aromatics into soups, stews, sauces, and stir-fries adds complexity and richness to dishes.

Umami-Boosting Ingredients

Umami-rich ingredients such as mushrooms, tomatoes, soy sauce, miso paste, and nutritional yeast add savory depth and richness to dishes. Incorporating umami-boosting ingredients into recipes enhances flavor and creates a satisfying taste experience. Umami-rich foods can be used in soups, sauces, marinades, and grain bowls to elevate the overall taste.

Homemade Spice Blends

Creating homemade spice blends allows individuals to customize flavor profiles and control the ingredients used. Mixing together a variety of herbs, spices, and aromatics enables individuals to create unique seasoning blends tailored to their taste preferences. Homemade spice blends can be used to season meats, vegetables, grains, and legumes, adding depth and complexity to dishes.

Chapter 7. Shopping Guide and Ingredient Substitutions

Smart Grocery Shopping Tips

Before heading to the grocery store, take time to plan your meals for the week. Create a detailed meal plan, including breakfasts, lunches, dinners, and snacks, based on your dietary preferences and nutritional goals. Check your pantry, refrigerator, and freezer to take stock of ingredients you already have and make a shopping list of items you need to purchase.

Stick to Your Shopping List

Once you've created a shopping list, stick to it while at the store to avoid impulse purchases. Shopping with a list helps you stay focused and ensures you only buy what you need. Resist the temptation to stray from your list by avoiding aisles or sections of the store where you're likely to encounter tempting but unnecessary items.

Shop the Perimeter of the Store

The perimeter of the grocery store typically contains fresh produce, meat, dairy, and other whole foods. Start your shopping trip by exploring the perimeter of the store first, focusing on nutrient-dense, whole foods that align with the principles of the Blood Type Diet. This strategy helps you prioritize fresh, minimally processed foods and avoid heavily processed or packaged items found in the center aisles.

Read Food Labels Carefully

When selecting packaged foods, take the time to read food labels carefully to assess their nutritional content and ingredients. Pay attention to serving sizes, calories, macronutrient breakdowns, and the presence of additives, preservatives, and artificial ingredients. Choose products with simple, recognizable ingredients and minimal added sugars, sodium, and unhealthy fats.

Choose Seasonal and Local Produce

Opt for seasonal fruits and vegetables whenever possible, as they tend to be fresher, more flavorful, and more affordable than out-of-season produce. Additionally, consider purchasing locally grown produce from farmers' markets or community-supported agriculture (CSA) programs to support local farmers and reduce your carbon footprint.

Stock Up on Staples

Keep your pantry stocked with essential staples that form the foundation of your meals on the Blood Type Diet. These staples may include whole grains, legumes, nuts, seeds, healthy oils, herbs, spices, and condiments. By having these items on hand, you can easily whip up nutritious meals and snacks without having to make frequent trips to the store.

Compare Prices and Look for Sales

Compare prices between brands and store brands to ensure you're getting the best value for your money. Look for sales, discounts, and promotions on staple items and stock up when prices are low. Consider purchasing non-perishable items in bulk to save money in the long run, but be mindful of storage space and expiration dates.

Avoid Shopping When Hungry

Shopping on an empty stomach can lead to impulse purchases and unhealthy food choices. Eat a balanced meal or snack before heading to the grocery store to curb cravings and make more rational decisions. Shopping with a satisfied stomach helps you stay focused on your shopping list and avoid succumbing to unhealthy temptations.

Consider Convenience and Preparation Time

Take into account the convenience and preparation time required for different foods when planning your meals and shopping list. Choose items that fit your schedule and cooking preferences, whether it's pre-cut vegetables, pre-cooked grains, or ready-to-eat proteins. Balancing convenience with nutritional quality ensures you can prepare healthy meals efficiently, even on busy days.

Substituting Ingredients for Compatibility

Before making ingredient substitutions, it's essential to understand the compatibility of certain foods with different blood types. For example, individuals with type A blood may thrive on a primarily plant-based diet, while those with type O blood may benefit from a higher intake of animal proteins. By familiarizing yourself with the recommended foods for your blood type, you can make informed substitutions that align with your dietary needs.

Protein Substitutions

For individuals following a plant-based diet or looking to reduce their intake of animal proteins, it's essential to identify suitable protein substitutes. Legumes such as beans, lentils, and chickpeas are excellent sources of plant-based protein that can replace meat or poultry in recipes. Tofu, tempeh, and seitan are also versatile options for adding protein to vegetarian and vegan dishes.

Grain Substitutions

Grains play a significant role in many diets but may need to be substituted for certain blood types or dietary preferences. For individuals with type O blood, who may benefit from reducing gluten-containing grains, alternatives such as quinoa, rice, millet, and buckwheat can be used in place of wheat, barley, and rye. Similarly, individuals with type A blood may choose to prioritize whole grains such as brown rice, oats, and spelt over refined grains.

Dairy Substitutions

Dairy products may not be well-tolerated by individuals with certain blood types or lactose intolerance. Fortunately, there are numerous dairy alternatives available, including almond milk, soy milk, coconut milk, and oat milk, which can be used in place of cow's milk in recipes. Plant-based alternatives such as cashew cheese, coconut yogurt, and almond-based cream can also replace traditional dairy products in dishes.

Sweetener Substitutions

Refined sugars are often discouraged on the Blood Type Diet due to their negative effects on health. However, there are several natural sweeteners that can be used as alternatives, including honey, maple syrup, coconut sugar, and date syrup. These sweeteners provide sweetness while also offering additional nutrients and antioxidants compared to refined sugars.

Fat Substitutions

Healthy fats are an essential component of the Blood Type Diet and can be obtained from various sources such as avocados, nuts, seeds, and olive oil. When substituting fats in recipes, opt for heart-healthy options such as avocado oil, coconut oil, or nut butter in place of unhealthy fats like butter or margarine. These alternatives provide beneficial fats and contribute to the overall nutritional profile of the dish.

Allergen-Free Substitutions

Individuals with food allergies or intolerances may need to make additional substitutions to accommodate their dietary restrictions. For example, those with gluten allergies can use gluten-free flours such as almond flour, coconut flour, or rice flour in place of wheat flour in baking recipes. Similarly, individuals with nut allergies can use seed butters or sunflower seed flour as alternatives to nut-based ingredients.

Experimenting with Flavor Profiles

When substituting ingredients, don't be afraid to experiment with different flavor profiles and culinary techniques. Incorporating herbs, spices, aromatics, and umami-rich ingredients can enhance the taste and complexity of dishes, even when making substitutions. Get creative in the kitchen and embrace the opportunity to discover new flavors and textures in your favorite recipes.

Adjusting Texture and Consistency

Some ingredient substitutions may alter the texture or consistency of a dish, requiring adjustments to the cooking method or additional ingredients. For example, using almond flour instead of wheat flour in baking may result in a denser texture, requiring additional leavening agents or moisture to achieve the desired outcome. Be prepared to adapt recipes as needed to maintain the integrity of the dish.

Chapter 8. Importance of Physical Activity

Exercise plays a vital role in overall health and well-being, and individuals with Blood Type A+ can benefit from incorporating specific types of physical activity into their routine. Tailoring exercise recommendations to complement the Blood Type Diet can enhance overall fitness levels, support weight management, and promote optimal health outcomes. Here are exercise recommendations specifically suited for individuals with Blood Type A+:

Gentle Aerobic Activities

Individuals with Blood Type A+ often respond well to gentle aerobic activities that promote relaxation and reduce stress levels. Engaging in activities such as walking, hiking, cycling, and swimming can help improve cardiovascular health, boost mood, and reduce anxiety. Aim for at least 30 minutes of moderate-intensity aerobic exercise most days of the week to reap the benefits of improved fitness and overall well-being.

Yoga and Tai Chi

Yoga and Tai Chi are excellent forms of exercise for individuals with Blood Type A+ due to their focus on mindfulness, flexibility, and stress reduction. These mind-body practices incorporate gentle movements, deep breathing techniques, and meditation to promote physical and mental relaxation. Practicing yoga or Tai Chi regularly can improve flexibility, balance, and posture while reducing muscle tension and promoting a sense of calm and well-being.

Pilates

Pilates is another low-impact exercise option that is well-suited for individuals with Blood Type A+. This form of exercise focuses on core strength, flexibility, and body awareness, making it an excellent choice for improving posture, stability, and muscle tone. Pilates exercises can be modified to accommodate different fitness levels and abilities, making it accessible to individuals of all ages and fitness backgrounds.

Mindful Movement Practices

In addition to structured exercise routines, individuals with Blood Type A+ can benefit from incorporating mindful movement practices into their daily lives. Activities such as gardening, dancing, and gentle stretching can promote physical activity while reducing stress and promoting relaxation. Practicing mindfulness during movement can enhance the mind-body connection and foster a sense of well-being.

Strength Training

While individuals with Blood Type A+ may not gravitate towards high-intensity strength training, incorporating light resistance exercises can still be beneficial for overall health and fitness. Using resistance bands, bodyweight exercises, or light weights can help maintain muscle tone, improve bone density, and support joint health. Aim to include strength training exercises 2-3 times per week, focusing on all major muscle groups.

Group Exercise Classes

Group exercise classes can provide social support, motivation, and variety to individuals with Blood Type A+. Choose classes that emphasize low-impact activities such as gentle yoga, Pilates, or group walking sessions. Group exercise classes can offer a sense of community and camaraderie while providing a structured environment for physical activity.

Outdoor Activities

Spending time outdoors in nature can enhance the benefits of exercise for individuals with Blood Type A+. Engage in activities such as hiking, nature walks, or outdoor yoga sessions to reap the physical and mental health benefits of being in natural surroundings. Connecting with nature can reduce stress, boost mood, and improve overall sense of well-being.

3-week Exercise Sample Plan

Week 1

Day 1: Gentle Yoga - Start the week with a gentle yoga session focusing on stretching and relaxation. Choose poses that promote flexibility and stress relief, such as Child's Pose, Cat-Cow, and Forward Fold.

Day 2: Brisk Walking - Enjoy a brisk walk outdoors for 30-45 minutes. Focus on maintaining a steady pace and incorporating natural scenery to uplift your spirits.

Day 3: Bodyweight Strength Training - Perform bodyweight exercises such as squats, lunges, push-ups, and planks for 20-30 minutes. Aim for 2-3 sets of 10-15 repetitions for each exercise.

Day 4: Rest or Active Recovery - Take a rest day or engage in light activities such as gentle stretching, foam rolling, or restorative yoga to promote recovery and relaxation.

Day 5: Pilates - Try a Pilates workout focusing on core strength and stability. Pilates exercises help improve posture, balance, and overall body awareness.

Day 6: Hiking or Nature Walk - Explore nature by going for a hike or nature walk in a scenic area. Choose a trail with varying terrain to challenge your muscles and immerse yourself in the beauty of the outdoors.

Day 7: Active Rest Day - Engage in low-impact activities such as swimming, cycling, or leisurely walking to keep your body moving while allowing for recovery.

Week 2

Day 8: Vinyasa Flow Yoga - Energize your body with a Vinyasa flow yoga class. Flow through dynamic sequences of poses linked with breath to build strength, flexibility, and mindfulness.

Day 9: Interval Training - Incorporate interval training into your workout routine by alternating between periods of high-intensity exercise (e.g., sprinting, jumping jacks) and recovery periods (e.g., walking or light jogging) for 20-30 minutes.

Day 10: Strength Training with Resistance Bands - Use resistance bands to perform strength-training exercises targeting major muscle groups. Resistance bands offer a versatile and effective way to build strength and improve muscle tone.

Day 11: Rest or Active Recovery - Take a rest day or engage in activities such as gentle yoga, foam rolling, or mobility exercises to aid in recovery and reduce muscle soreness.

Day 12: Dance Fitness Class - Have fun and burn calories with a dance fitness class such as Zumba or hip-hop dance. Dance workouts are a great way to boost cardiovascular health and improve coordination.

Day 13: Outdoor Recreation - Spend time outdoors engaging in recreational activities such as kayaking, paddleboarding, or playing frisbee. Enjoy the sunshine and fresh air while staying active.

Day 14: Active Rest Day - Participate in leisurely activities such as gardening, leisurely cycling, or playing with pets to keep your body moving and promote relaxation.

Week 3

Day 15: Mindful Movement - Practice mindful movement with activities such as Tai Chi or Qigong. These gentle forms of exercise focus on slow, deliberate movements to promote relaxation, balance, and mental clarity.

Day 16: Circuit Training - Create a circuit workout incorporating a variety of exercises such as jumping jacks, burpees, mountain climbers, and bicycle crunches. Perform each exercise for 30-60 seconds with minimal rest between exercises.

Day 17: Functional Training - Incorporate functional exercises that mimic everyday movements, such as squats, lunges, and overhead presses. Focus on improving strength, stability, and mobility to enhance overall functional fitness.

Day 18: Rest or Active Recovery - Take a rest day or engage in activities such as gentle stretching, foam rolling, or restorative yoga to support muscle recovery and relaxation.

Day 19: Indoor Cycling - Enjoy a high-energy indoor cycling class to improve cardiovascular endurance and lower-body strength. Follow along with an instructor-led class or create your own playlist for a personalized workout.

Day 20: Circuit Training - Repeat the circuit training workout from Day 16, focusing on maintaining proper form and challenging yourself with increased intensity or resistance.

Day 21: Active Rest Day - Engage in light activities such as leisurely walking, swimming, or playing recreational sports with friends and family to round out the week and keep your body moving while allowing for recovery.

Conclusion

In the journey towards balancing work, relationships, and self-care, it's crucial to recognize that achieving perfect equilibrium is a lofty ideal, often elusive in the face of life's unpredictability. Instead, it's about embracing the ebb and flow of these elements, finding harmony amidst the chaos, and prioritizing what truly matters to you. By setting boundaries, practicing self-care, and nurturing relationships, you create a foundation for resilience and well-being that allows you to navigate the challenges of daily life with greater ease.

At the heart of this balance lies the art of self-awareness – the ability to recognize your own needs, limitations, and desires, and to honor them with compassion and understanding. Self-awareness empowers you to make conscious choices that align with your values and priorities, leading to a more fulfilling and authentic way of living. It's about listening to your inner voice, trusting your intuition, and honoring the wisdom that resides within you.

As you cultivate balance in your life, remember the importance of flexibility and adaptability. Life is full of unexpected twists and turns, and rigid adherence to a predetermined plan can lead to frustration and disappointment. Instead, embrace change as an opportunity for growth, learning, and self-discovery. Approach challenges with curiosity and resilience, knowing that every setback is a stepping stone on the path to greater wisdom and fulfillment.

Gratitude serves as a powerful antidote to the stresses and pressures of modern life, reminding us of the abundance and beauty that surround us each day. By cultivating gratitude for the blessings in your life – both big and small – you shift your focus from scarcity to abundance, from fear to appreciation. Gratitude opens your heart to joy, connection, and possibility, allowing you to savor the richness of life's experiences with humility and grace.

Finally, remember that balance is not a destination to be reached, but a journey to be embraced. It requires ongoing effort, patience, and self-reflection, as well as a willingness to course-correct when necessary. Be gentle with yourself as you navigate the complexities of balancing work, relationships, and self-care, and celebrate the progress you make along the way. Ultimately, the pursuit of balance is a deeply personal and transformative endeavor, guiding you towards a life of greater harmony, fulfillment, and meaning.